Title: *Emma and Jake share a secret*

Writer:: Siomara Yogini (Siomara Narváez).

Illustrations: Alejandra Huerga

Pages: 54

ISBN-13: 978-1547195473

ISBN-10: 1547195479

Genre: Education, Motivation, Yoga.

Year of Publication: 2017.

© **Of the Texts of the Book:** The Author.

Edition and design:
John Navidad
johnnavidadNY@gmail.com
www.manhattanboundbooks.com

Website: **www.siomarayogini.com**
Email: **beyou@siomarayogini.com**

Emma and Jake share a secret

A kids story to introduce the benefits of a Yoga Practice

Text: Siomara Yogini
Ilustrated by: Alejandra Huerga

This book is dedicated to the children who
have brightened my days since 2010
with their smiles, hugs, questions,
and unbelievable statements.

You are my inspiration and one of my greatest motivators!

My heart is full of deep gratitude...

Thank you to my wonderful parents.
Thank you to my unconditional sisters/friends.
Thank you to my teachers and guides.
Thank you to The Creative Energy that we called God.

I am but the result of a collection of experiences and events.
Thanks to all of you who were part of them.

Namaste!

This is the story of Emma and Jake, two
wonderful kids who meet one day
at summer camp.

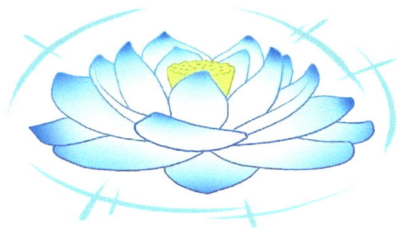

Jake is very smart and an adventurous kid.
He loves to explore and learn new things,
and is a superhero in his dreams.

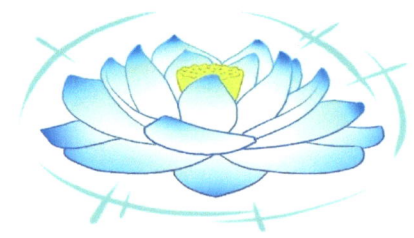

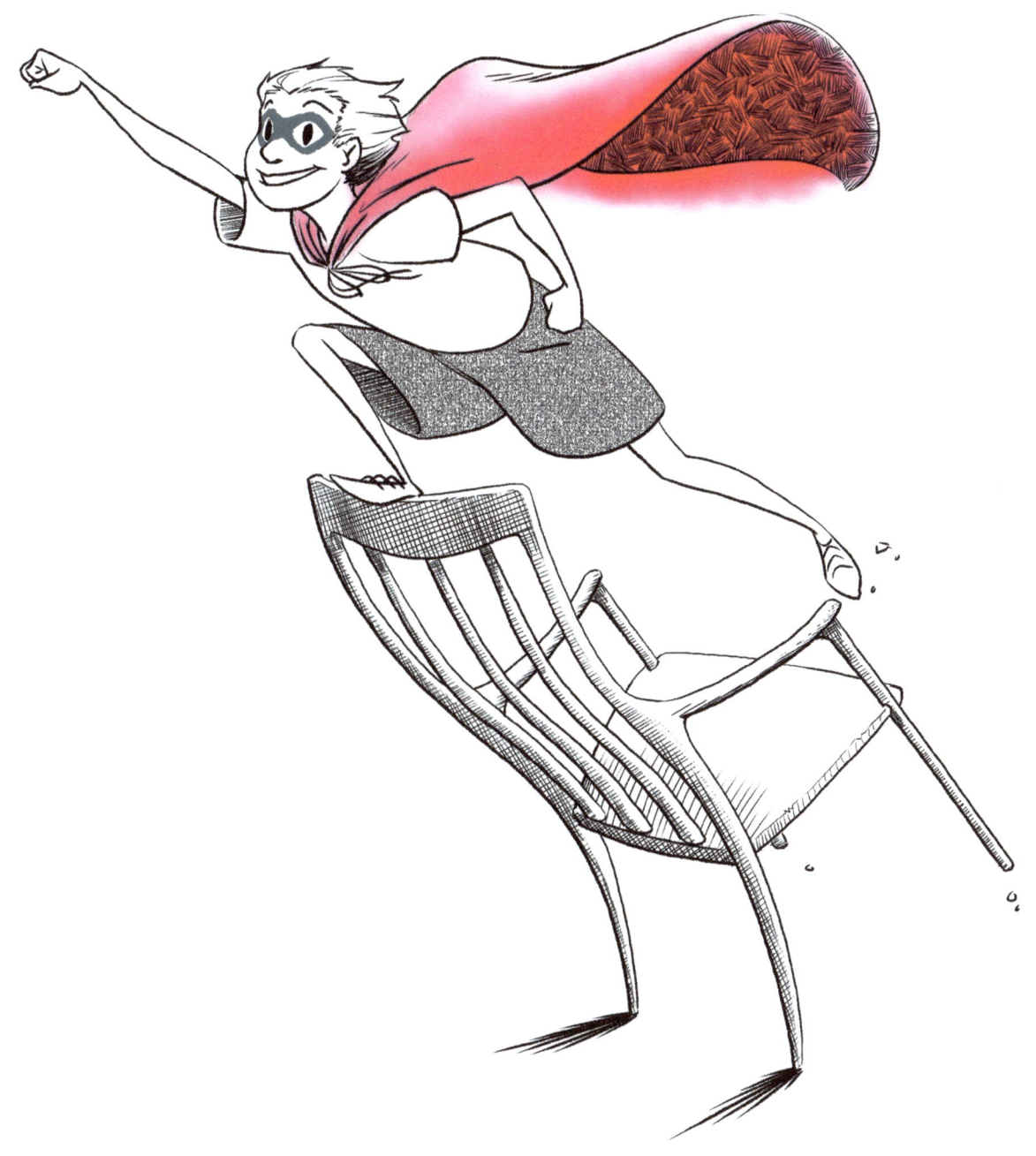

Sometimes, it is challenging for Jake to concentrate and focus at school.

Jake's mind is always wondering about the new places he could explore, the games he could play, and all the exciting things he could be doing.

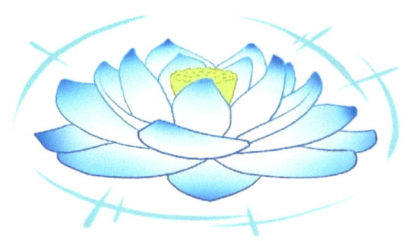

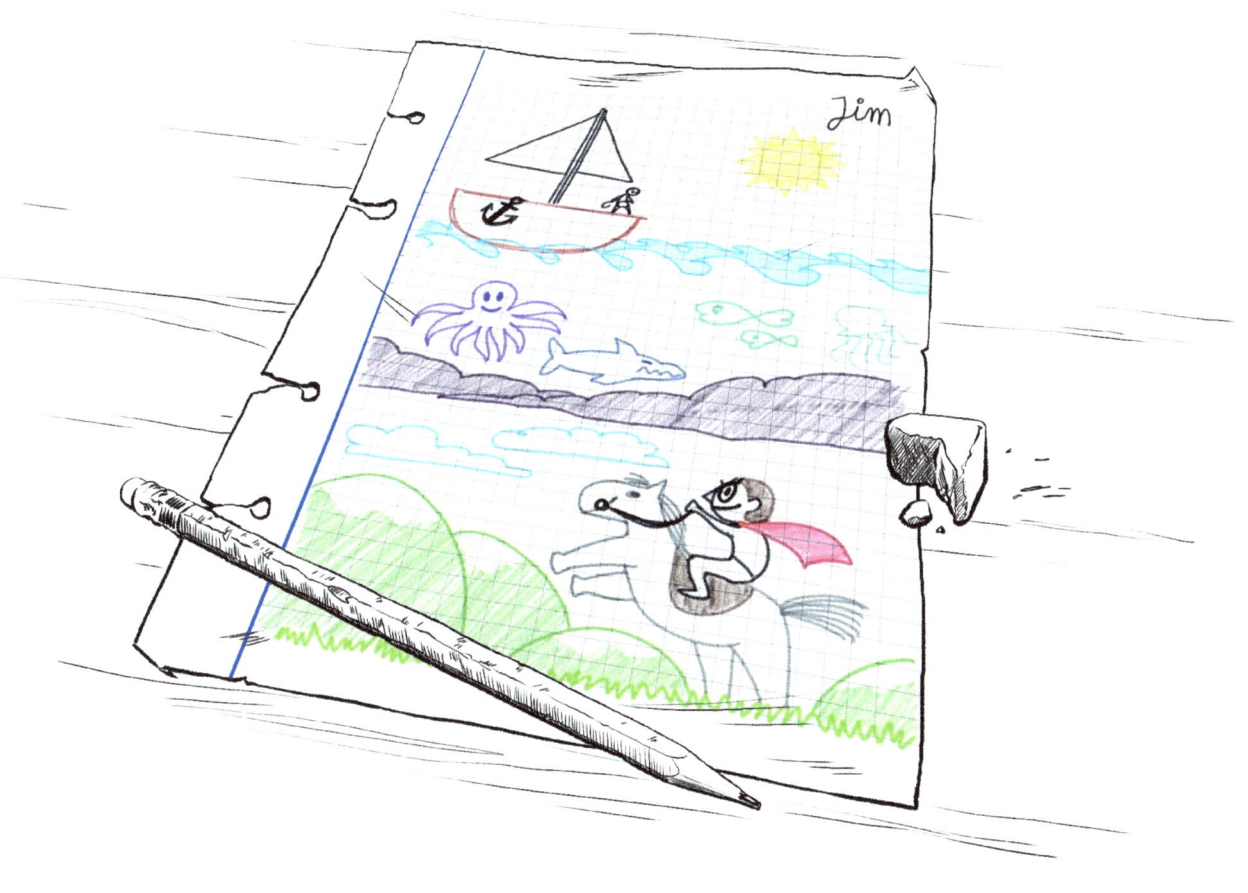

Emma is a joyful and creative girl who loves nature and feels free when dancing.

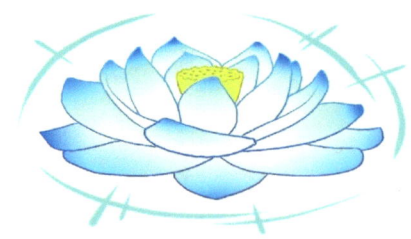

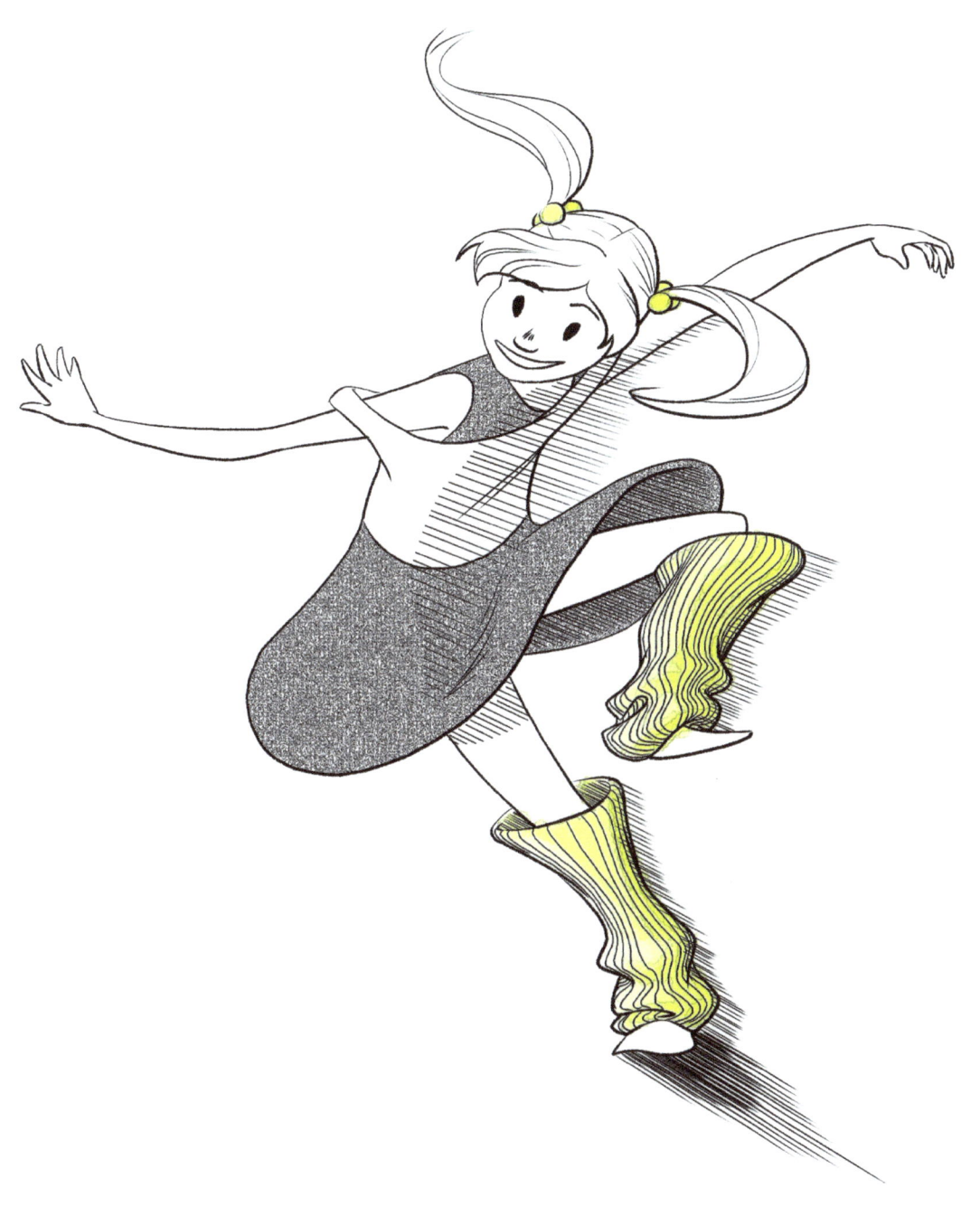

She used to have troubles at school too.

Emma used to spend her time daydreaming, playing and
having fun than paying attention to the lessons
given at school.
But, not anymore.

Emma knows a secret she will very soon share with Jake.

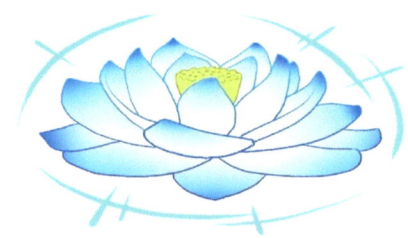

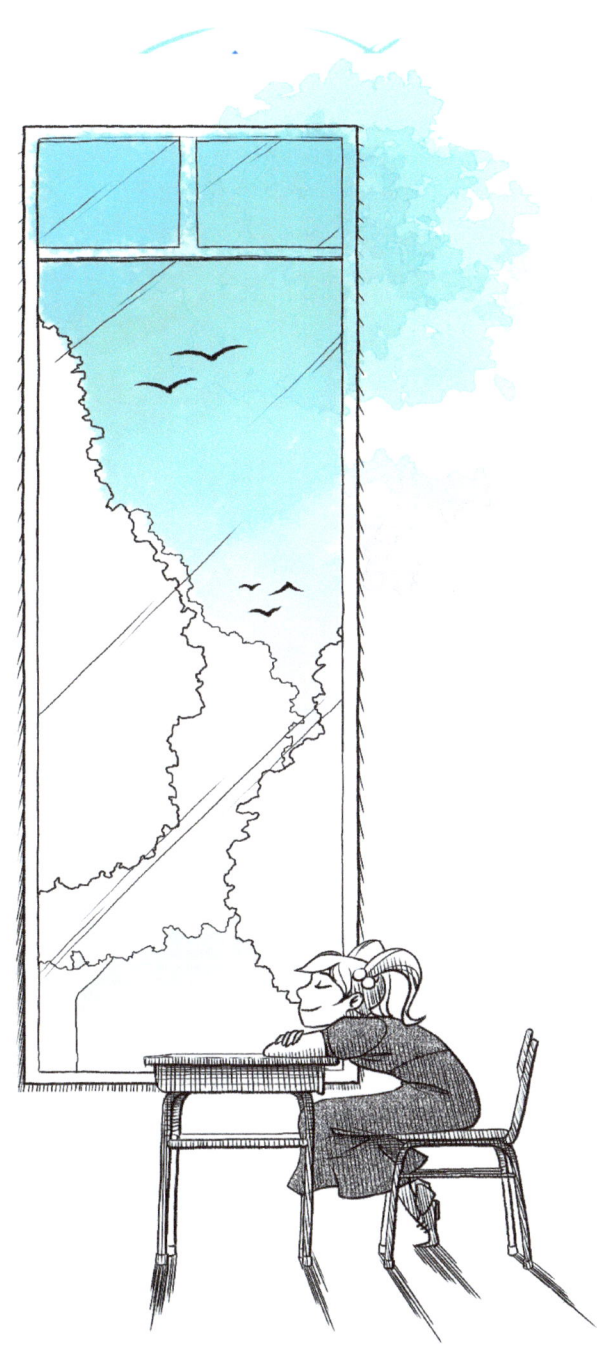

It is the first day of summer camp and there are children arriving from different cities. Jake gets off the bus full of excitement in seeing so many children, trees, birds and imagining all the new places to explore.

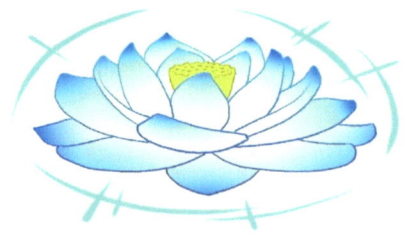

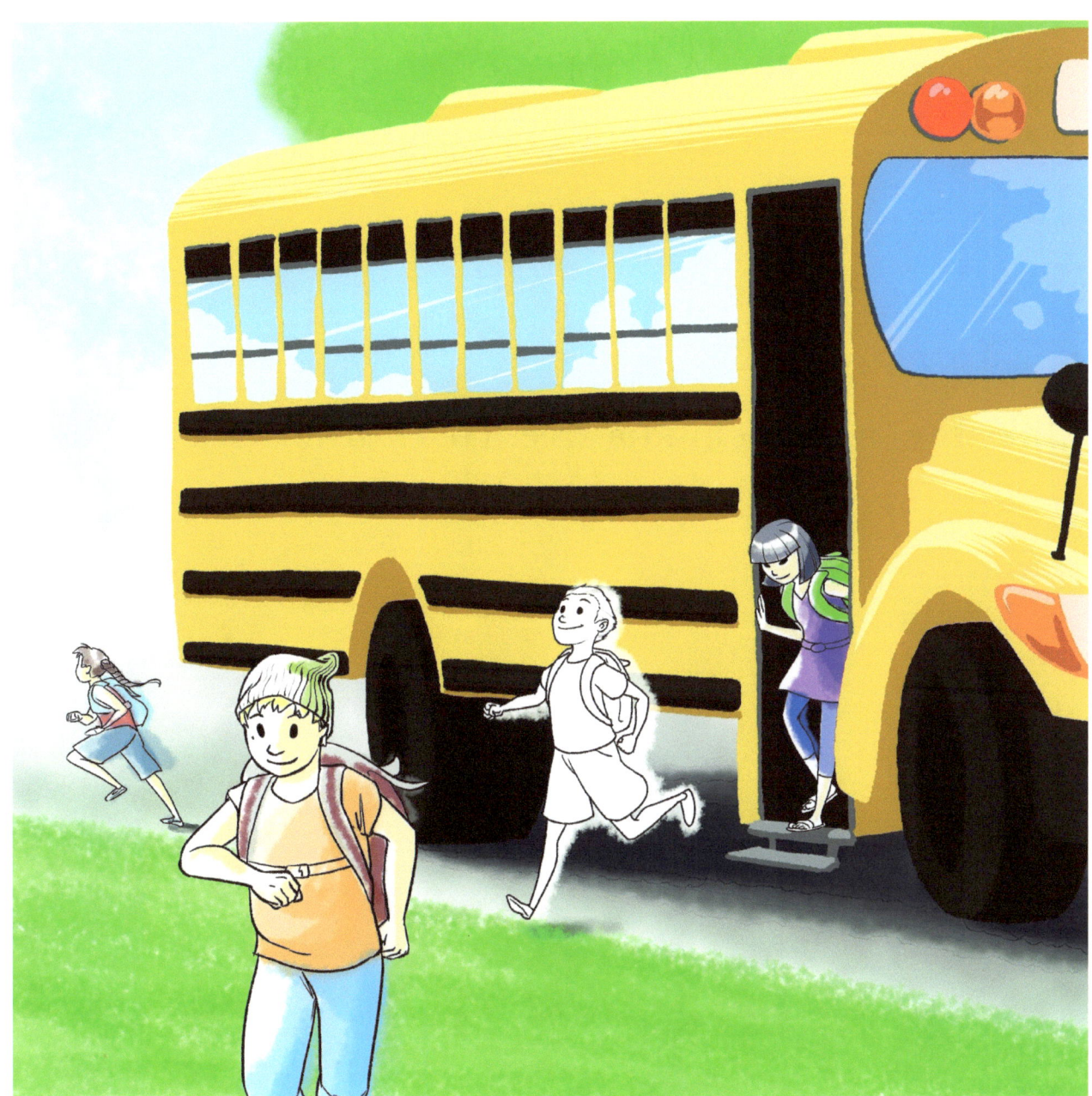

Jake sees a girl behind a tree. He throws a stick to her to draw her attention.

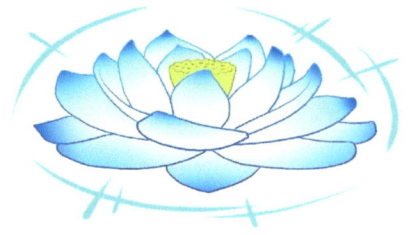

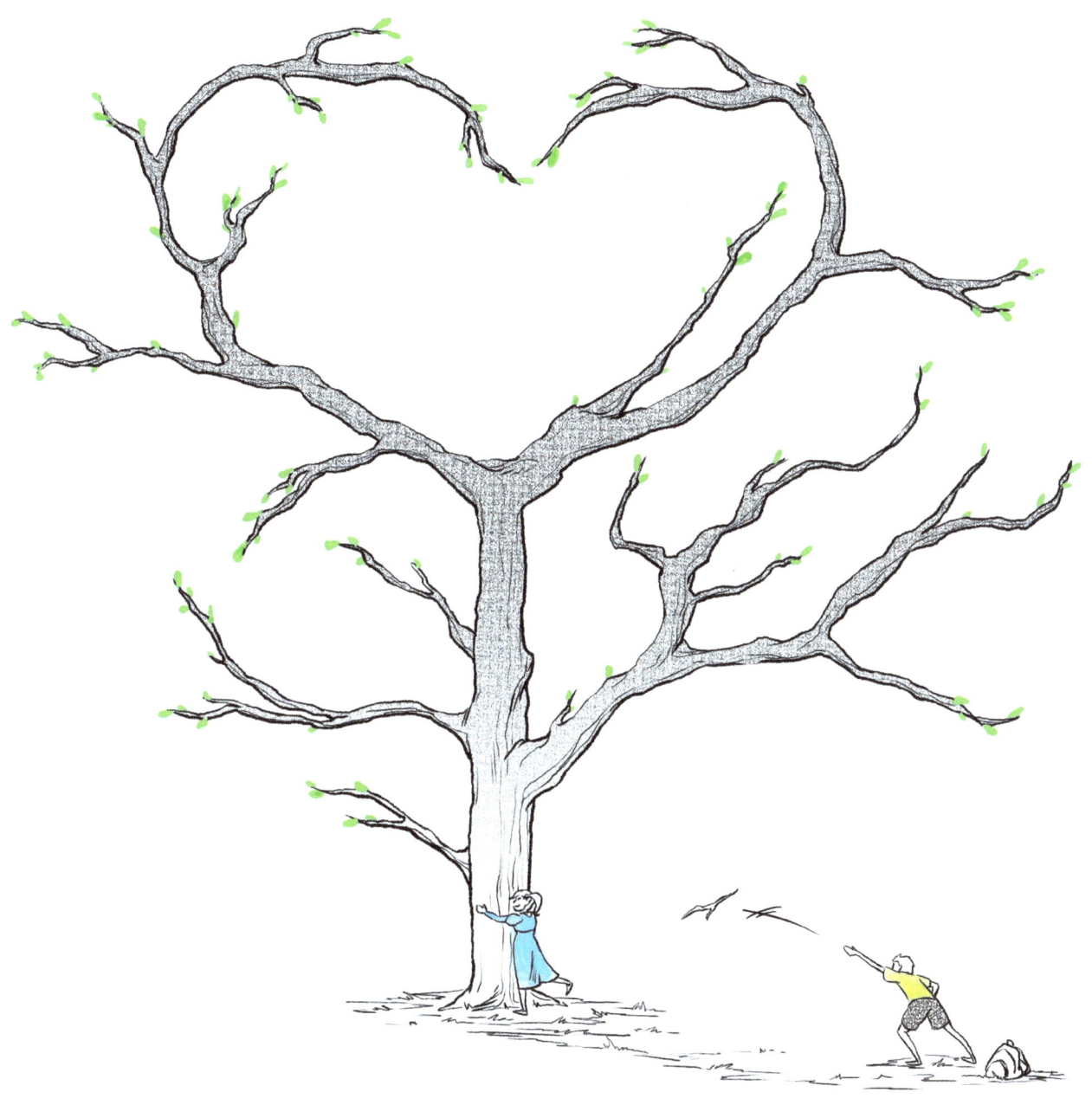

"Hey, what are you doing?" he asks.
"Hugging a tree, don't you see?"
"Hugging a tree? I prefer to climb on it…"
"Trees feel just like you and me".
"I agree."
"Let's go up the tree" Emma replies.

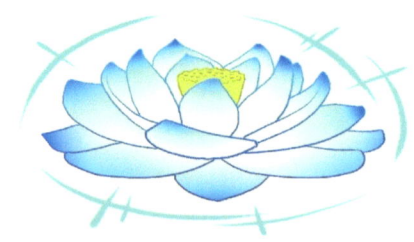

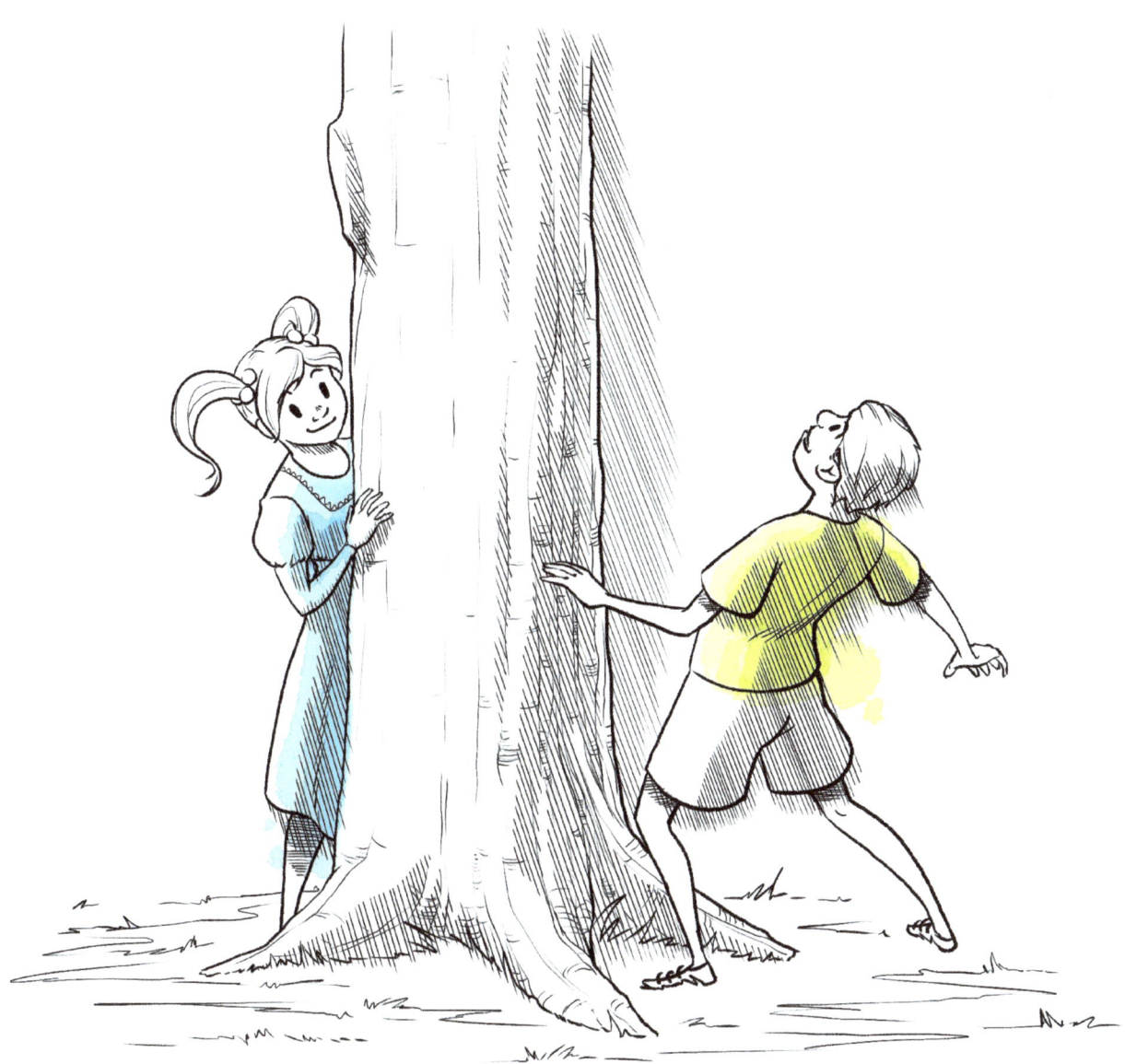

And so up and up the three they went. Emma and Jake played and giggled from branch to branch until someone shouted "dinner is ready!"

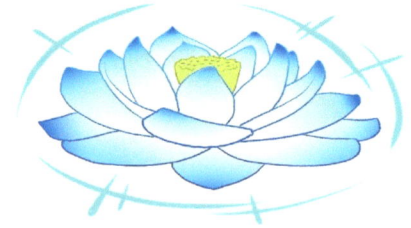

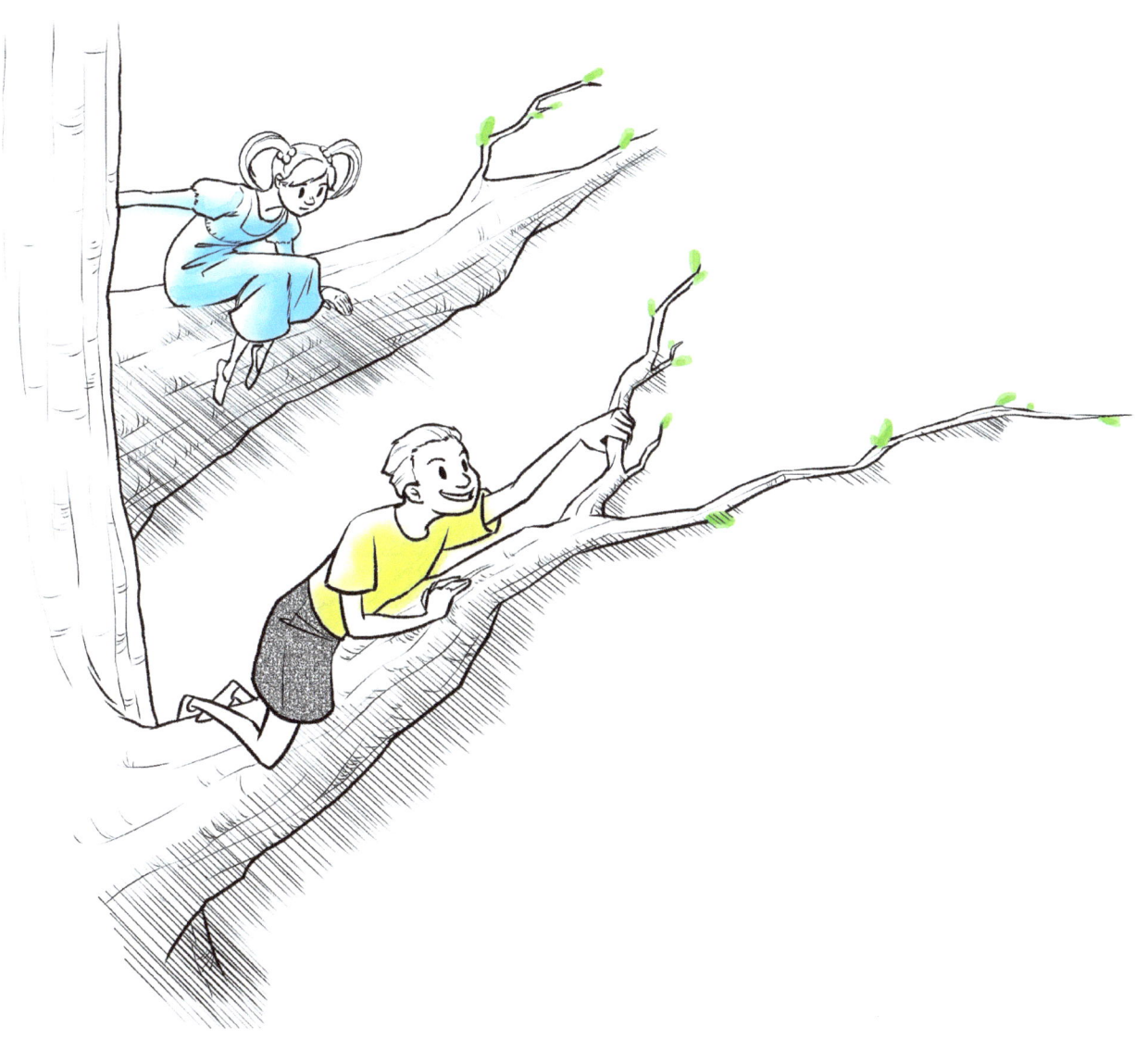

Emma and Jake rush down the tree.
Emma goes down first
but Jake falls right after her.

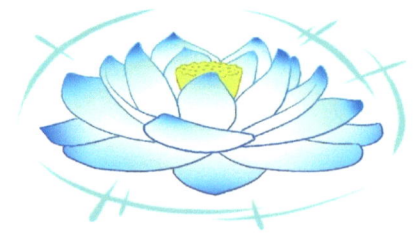

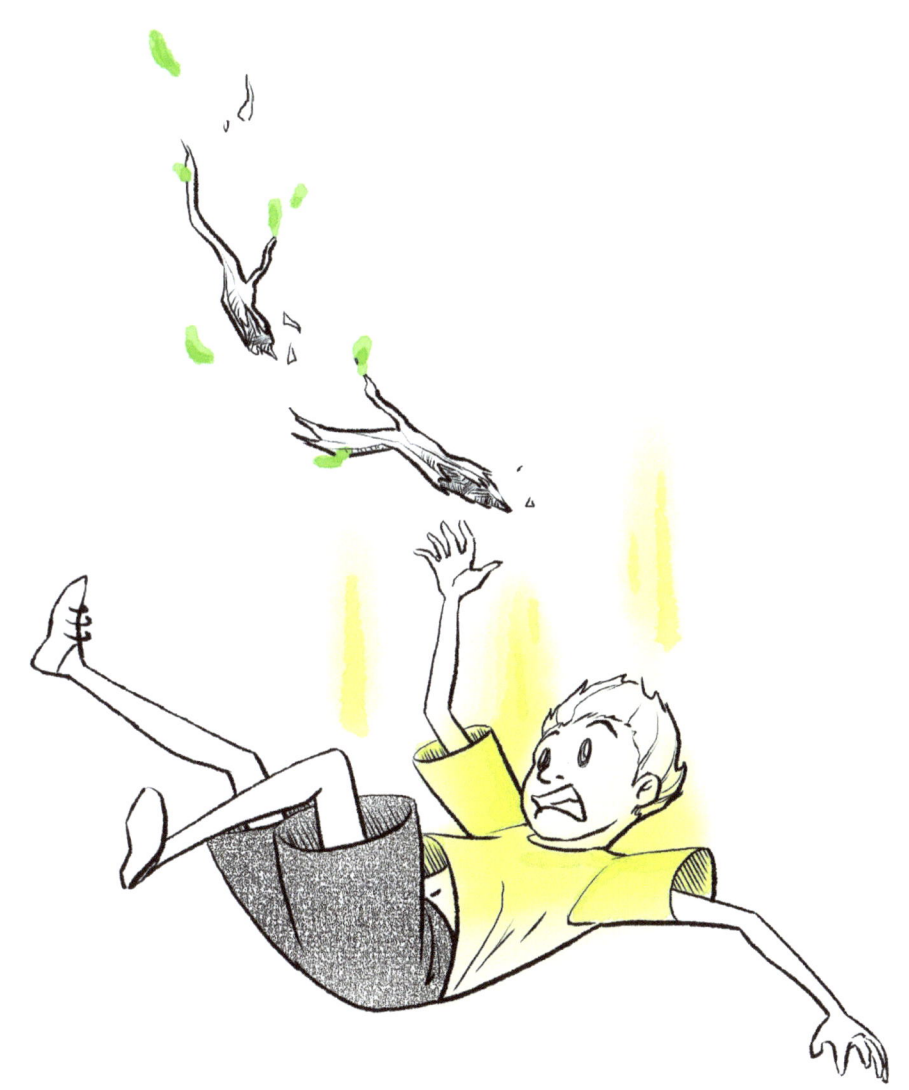

Jake scratches his knee and it starts to bleed.

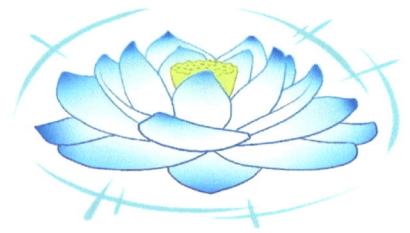

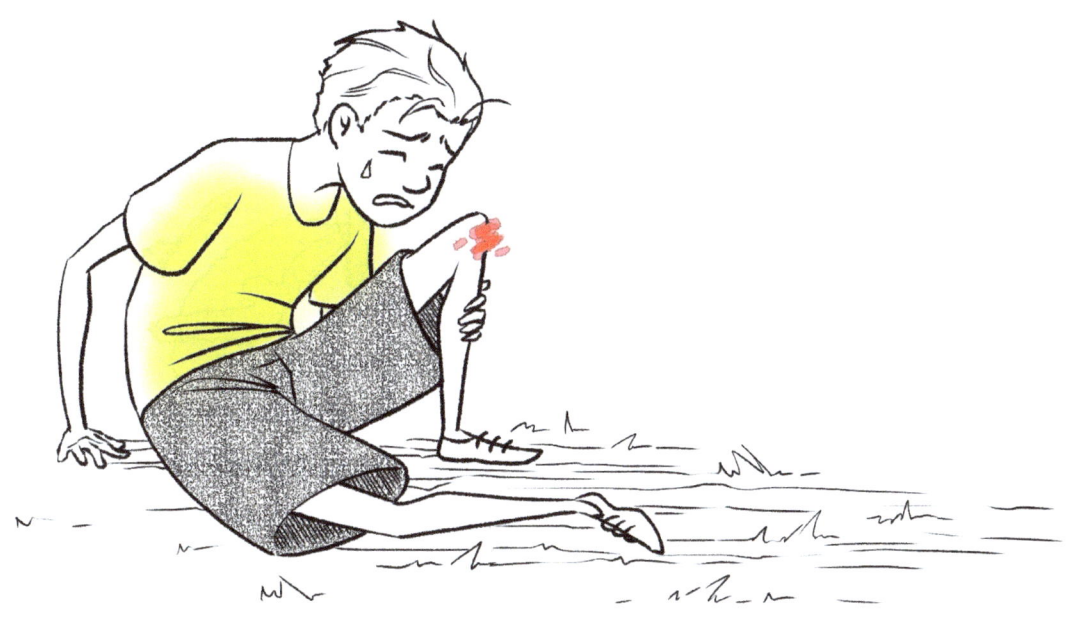

Jake is crying and Emma puts her hands
around his knee.
Emma closes her eyes and starts to breathe.

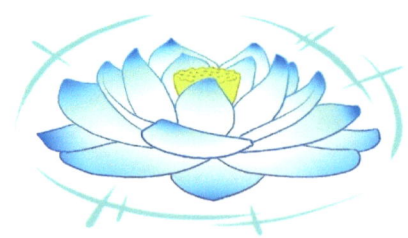

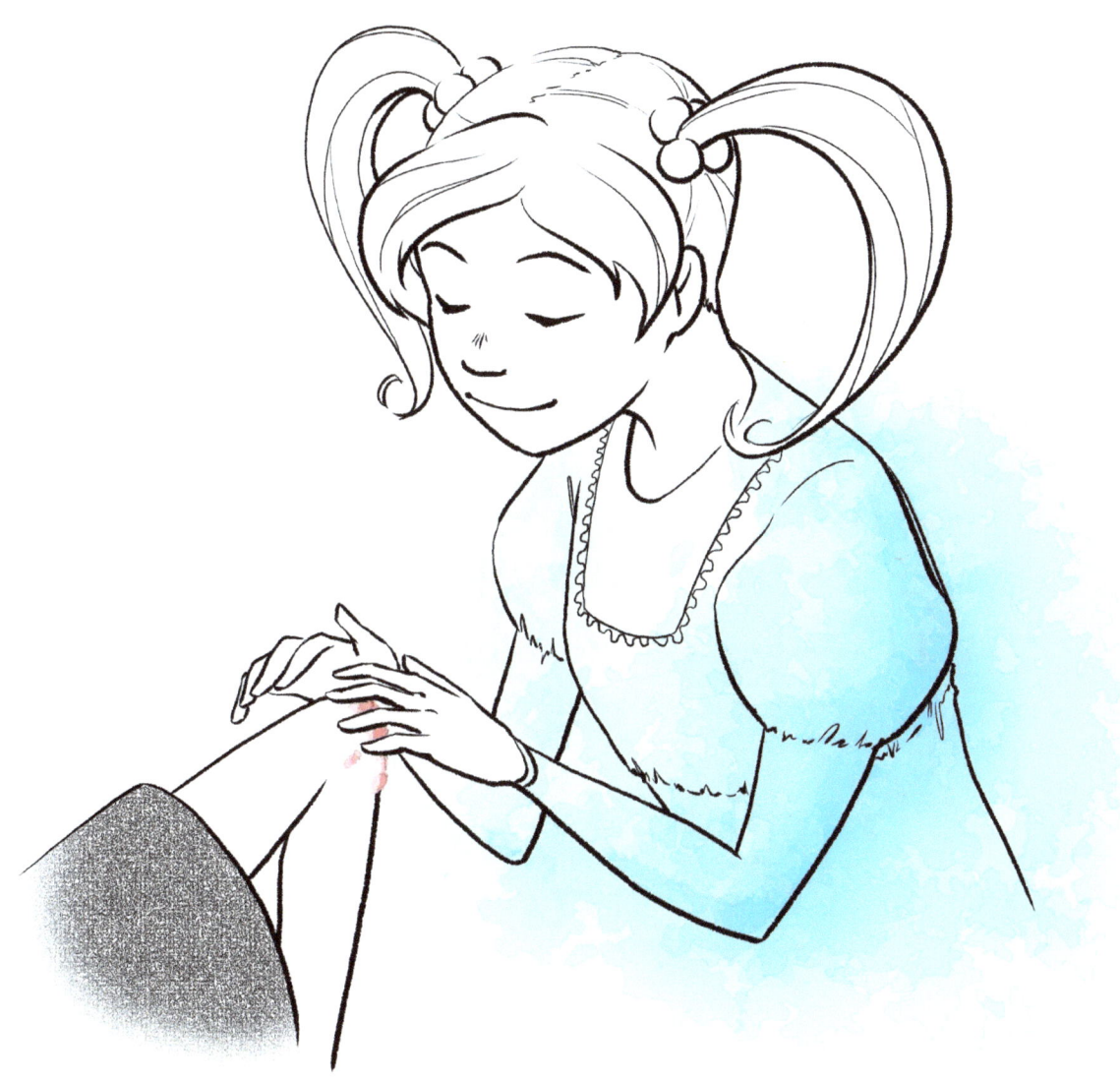

Jake is confused but he starts to feel a warm
sensation on his knee...
"What are you doing?" he asks.
"Oh, I am sending you good thoughts. This is called
the loving touch and you can do it with everyone
you love. Don't you feel better?" Emma responds.
"Yes! I do feel better.
I like the loving touch!" Jake says.

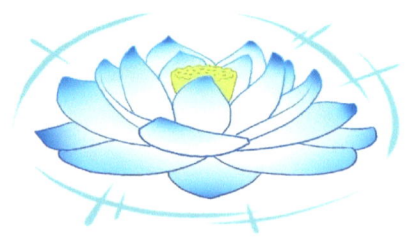

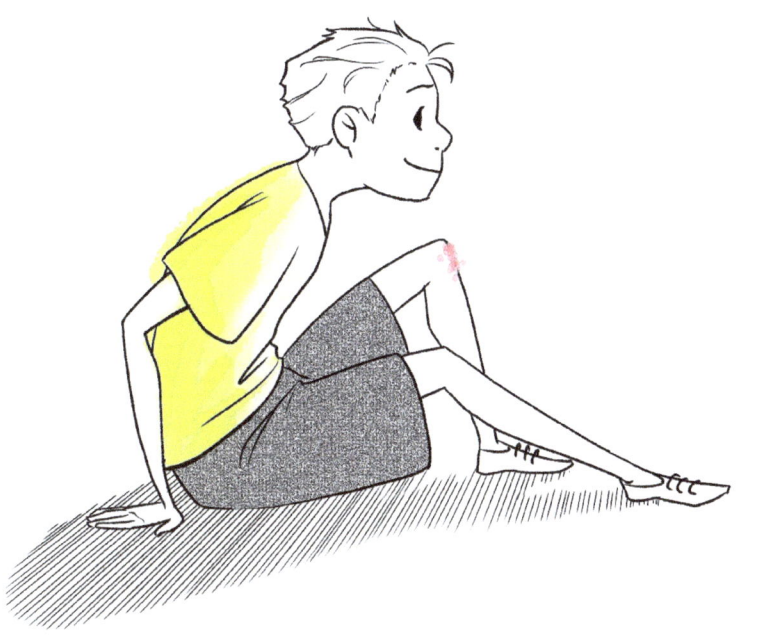
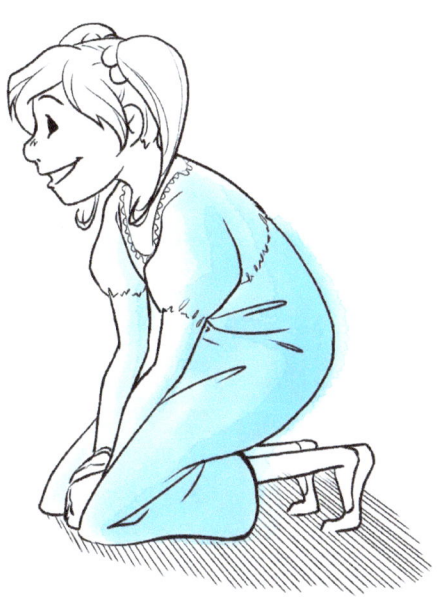

Emma and Jake say their goodbyes
for the night.

***

The next day, Emma is waiting for Jake under the tree
and wondering where he could be.

Emma is getting impatient so she decides to sit,
close her eyes and breathe.

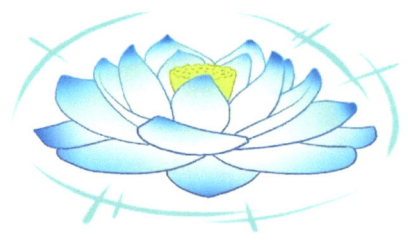

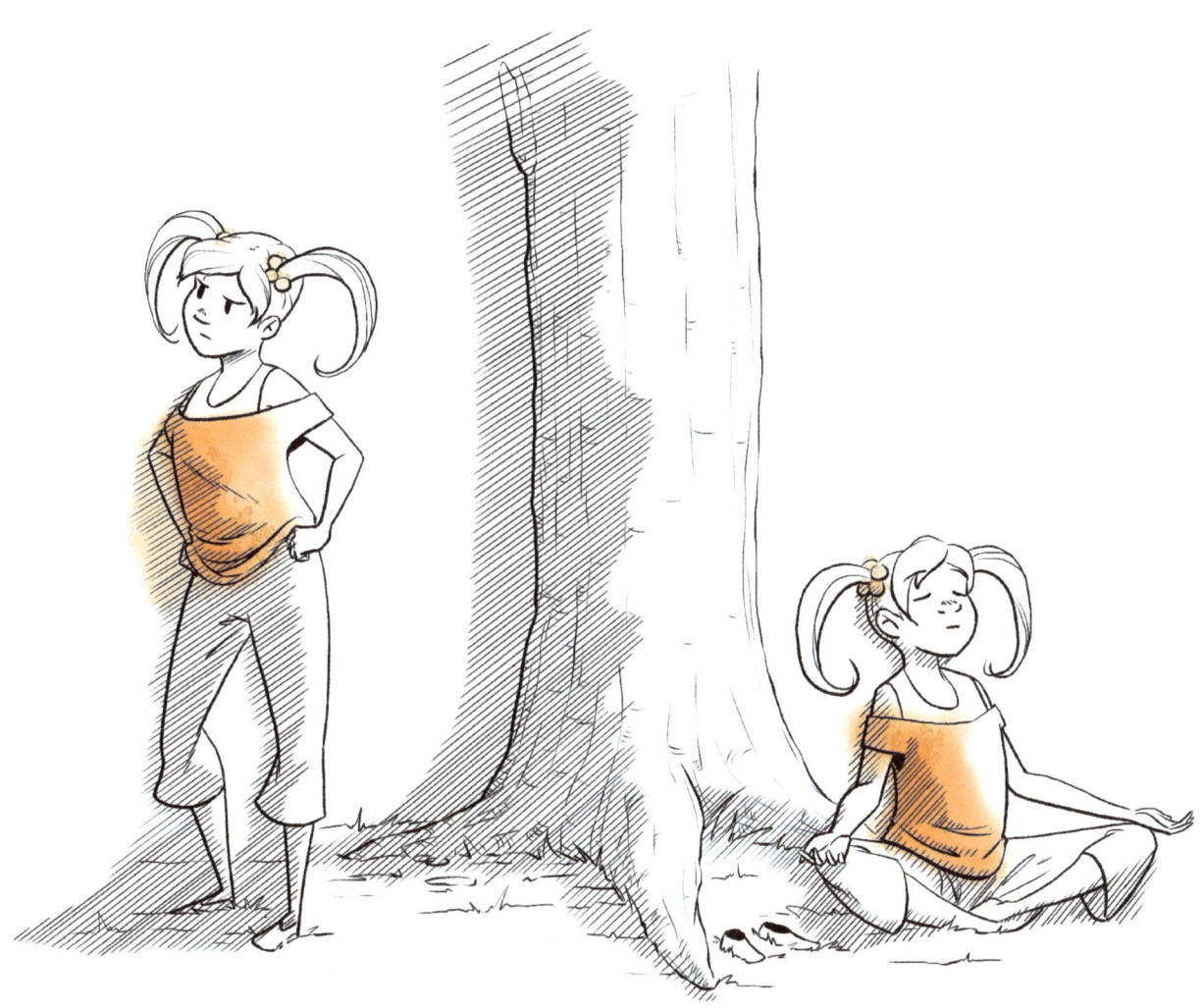

Jake comes running, tired, and panting like a dog.

"What happened, Jake, what took you
so long?" Emma asks.

"Oh, someone gave me an assignment but I was so
excited about going out that I didn't understand
what I was supposed to do and it took me a long time to
figure it out" Jake responds.

"Oh, Jake, I used to be just like you. It was hard for me
to pay attention and stay still but I learned an ancient
secret. It keeps me happy, healthy, and focused."

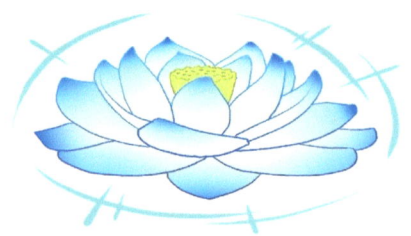

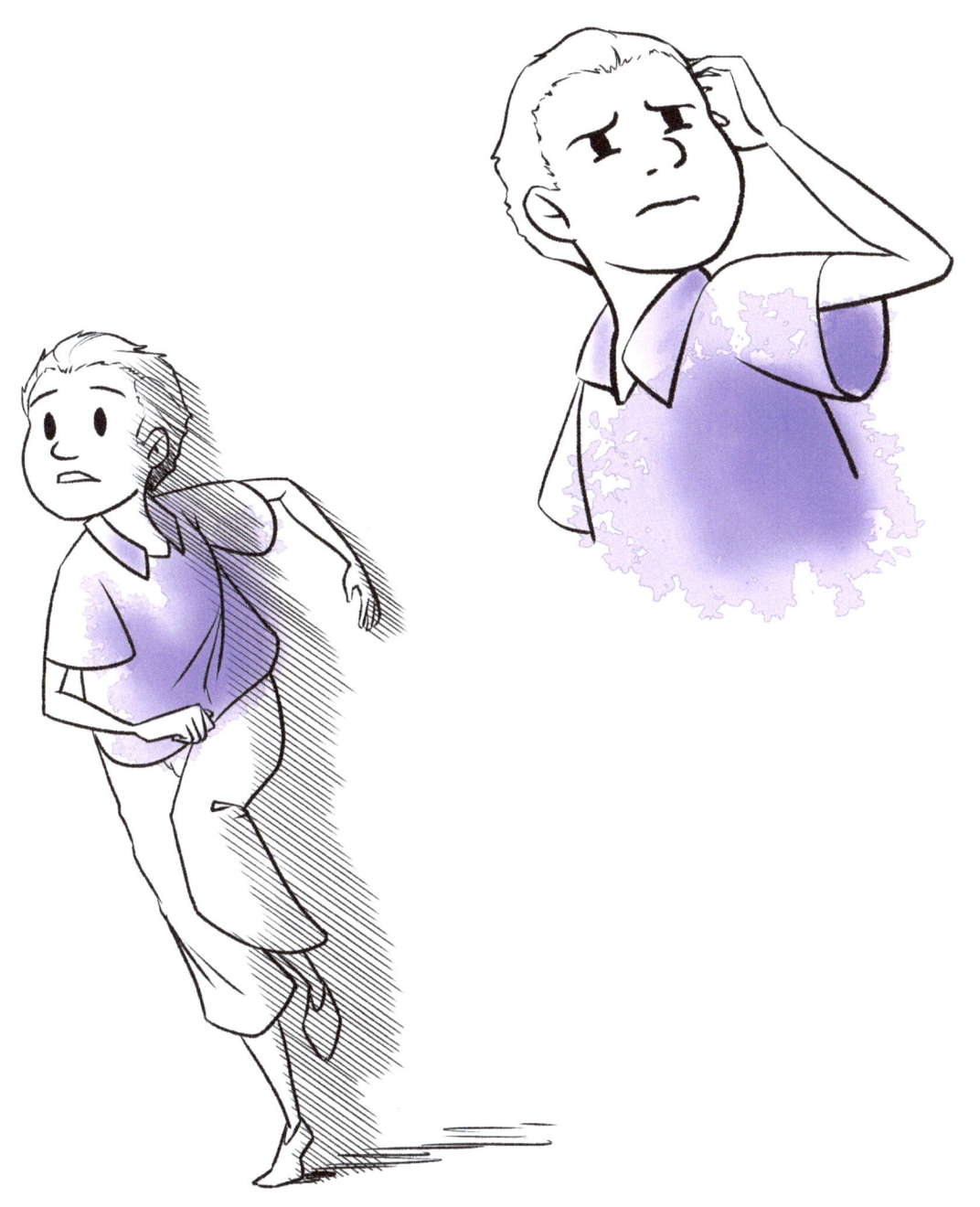

"The secret is to coordinate your movements with the breath. It is called Yoga. Let me show you: imagine you are a mountain standing peacefully and strong on your feet".

"Now while inhaling through your nose lift your arms to the sky as you salute the clouds and the sun. Feel the air touching your hair."

"It is time to greet Mother Earth... Exhale and touch the ground making an exhaling sound."

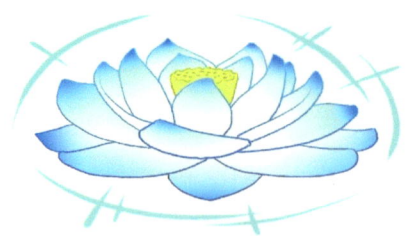

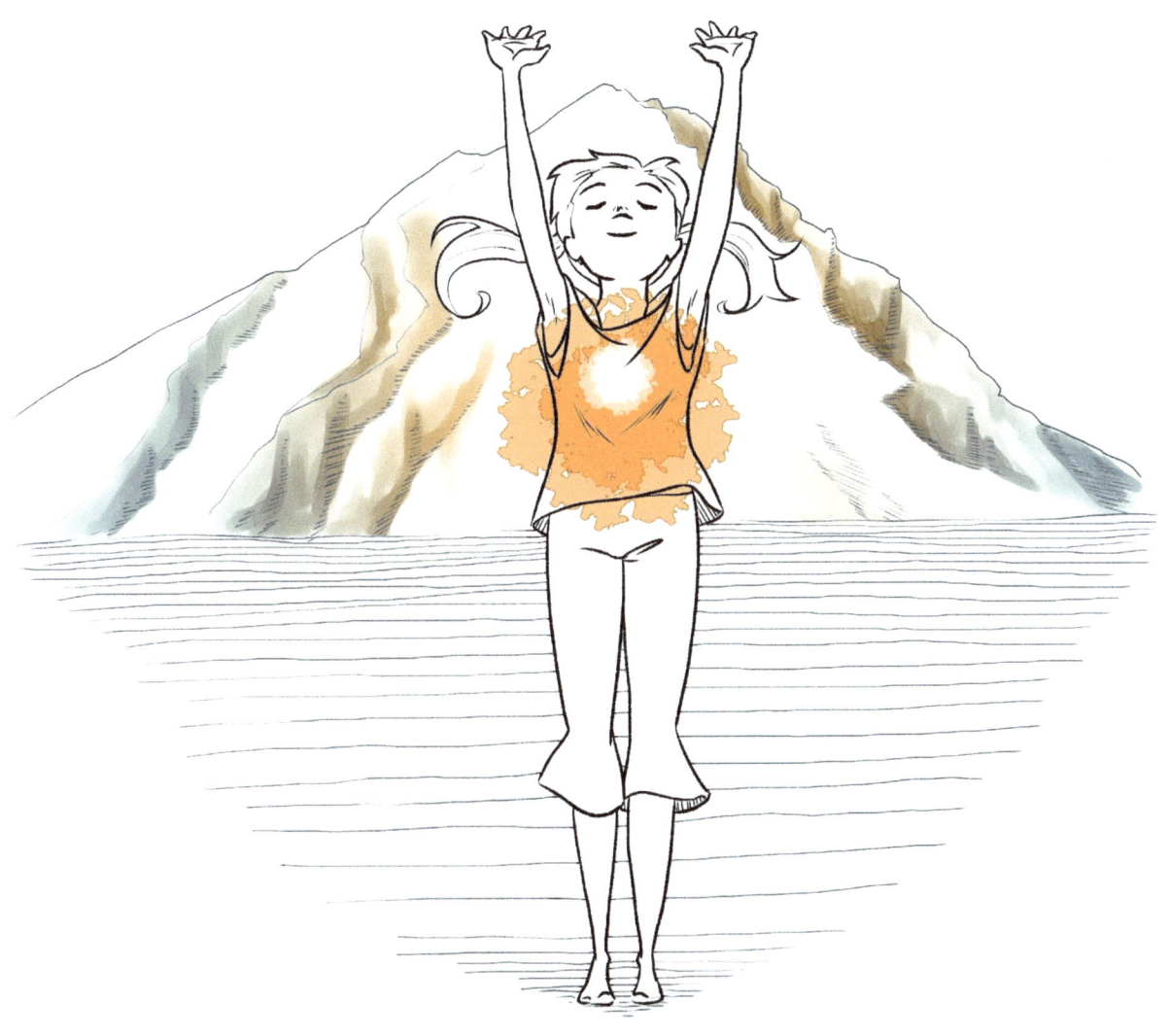

"Plant your hands on the floor. Inhale and jump your legs back in plank pose. Feel your legs and arms becoming stronger while you are humming OMMMMMM!!!"

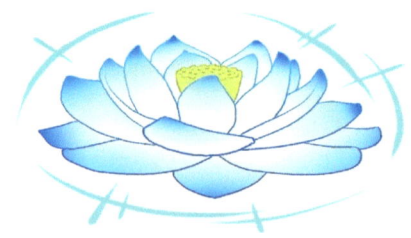

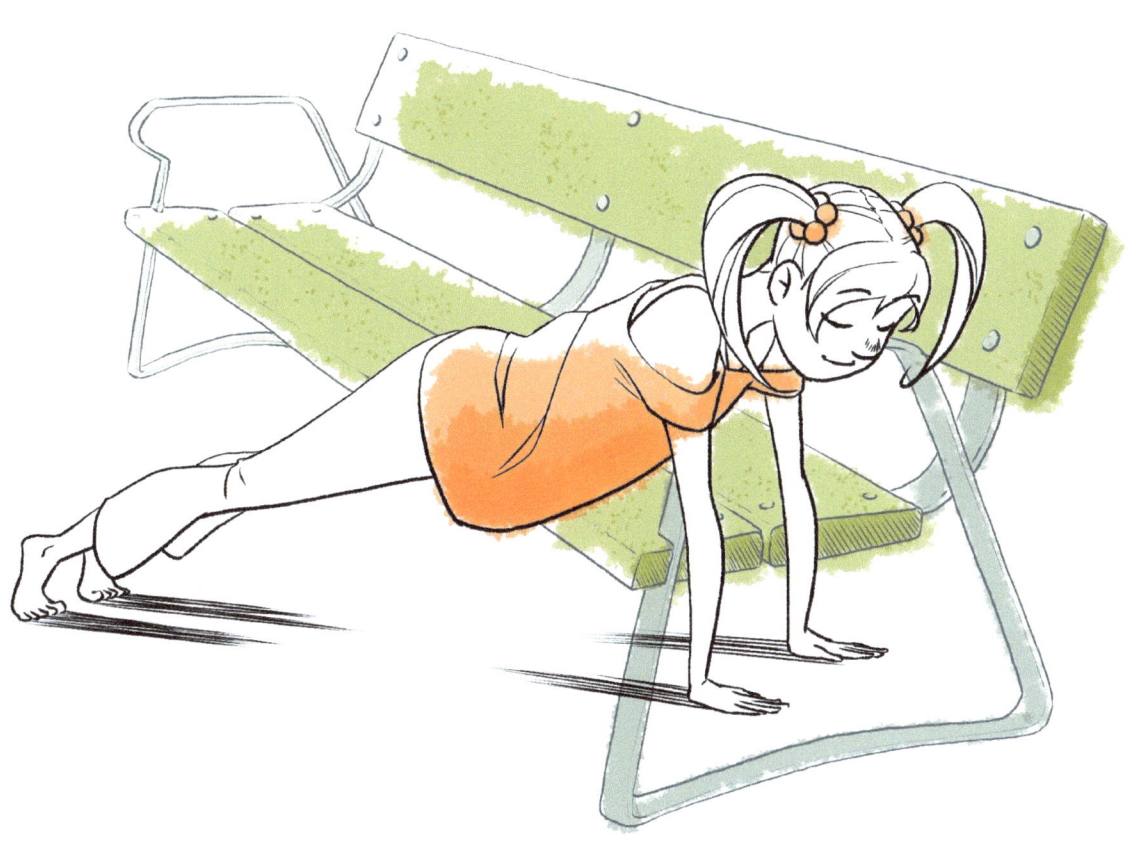

"Exhale bringing your body to the floor. Take a sip of air through your nose. It is time for cobra pose. Plant your hands and lift the chest. Smile with grace, it lights up your face."

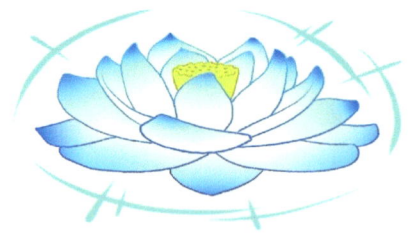

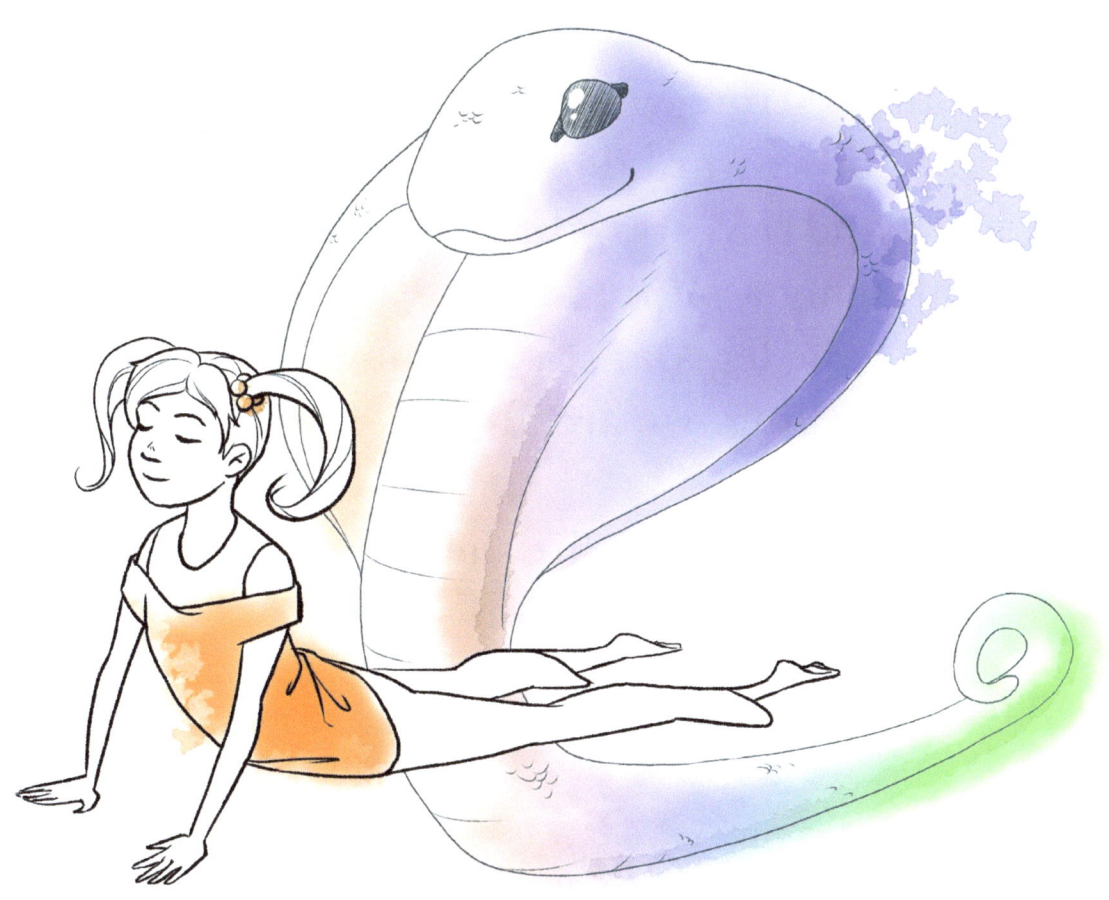

"It is time to be strong. As you exhale, push yourself back into downward dog. Your head is off the floor, arms and legs straight. You look great! Feel the joy of being a puppy, inhale and wiggle your tail. Lift one leg and stay strong. Just keep breathing, we are almost done."

"Don't forget to lift the other leg.
Don't worry if you sweat".

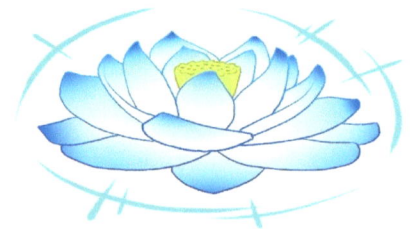

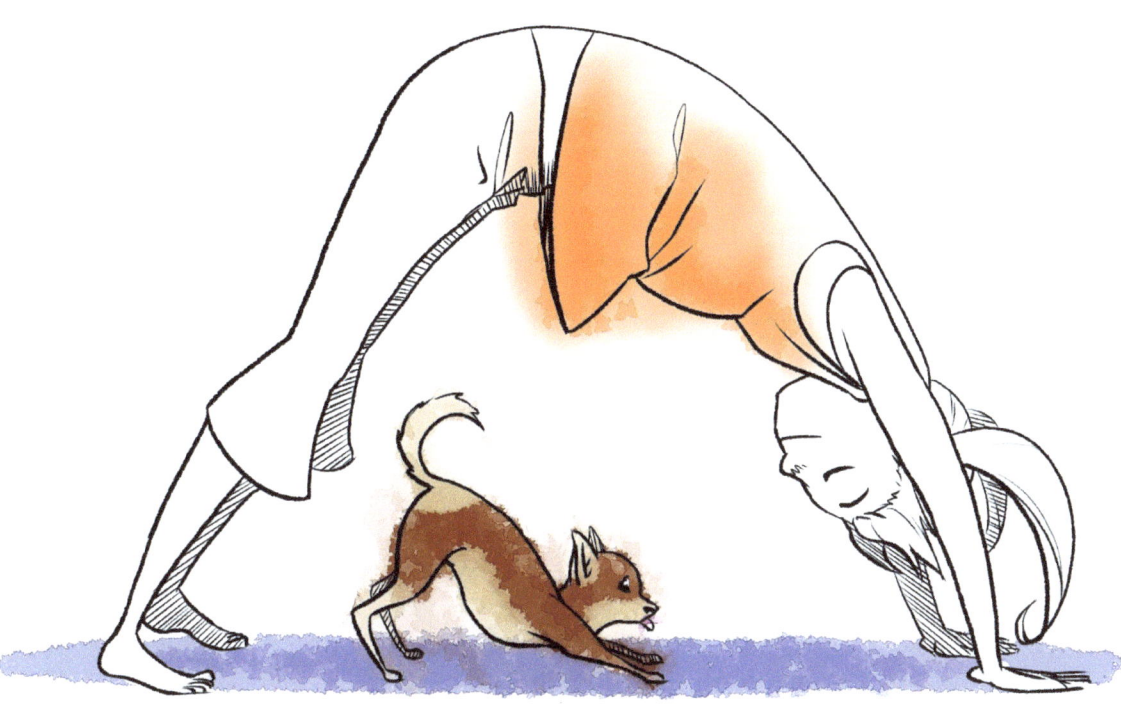

"Walk your feet to your hands.
Open your arms and take a deep breath in.
It's a beautiful day, be truthful with yourself.
Put the hands together over the head."

"Exhale and close your eyes. Bring your hands together in front of your heart. Yes, you can giggle, its ok to smile. Imagine you have roots. Feel your feet connected to the ground and dont make any sounds. Lift one foot and put it against the other leg.

Spread your branches over the head. Stand strong. It won't be too long. You are on tree pose."

"Change legs and grow again. If you keep falling, try again."

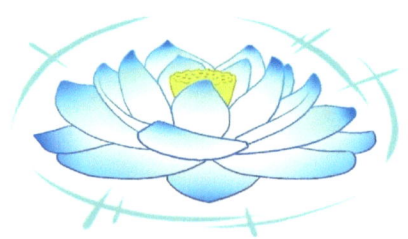

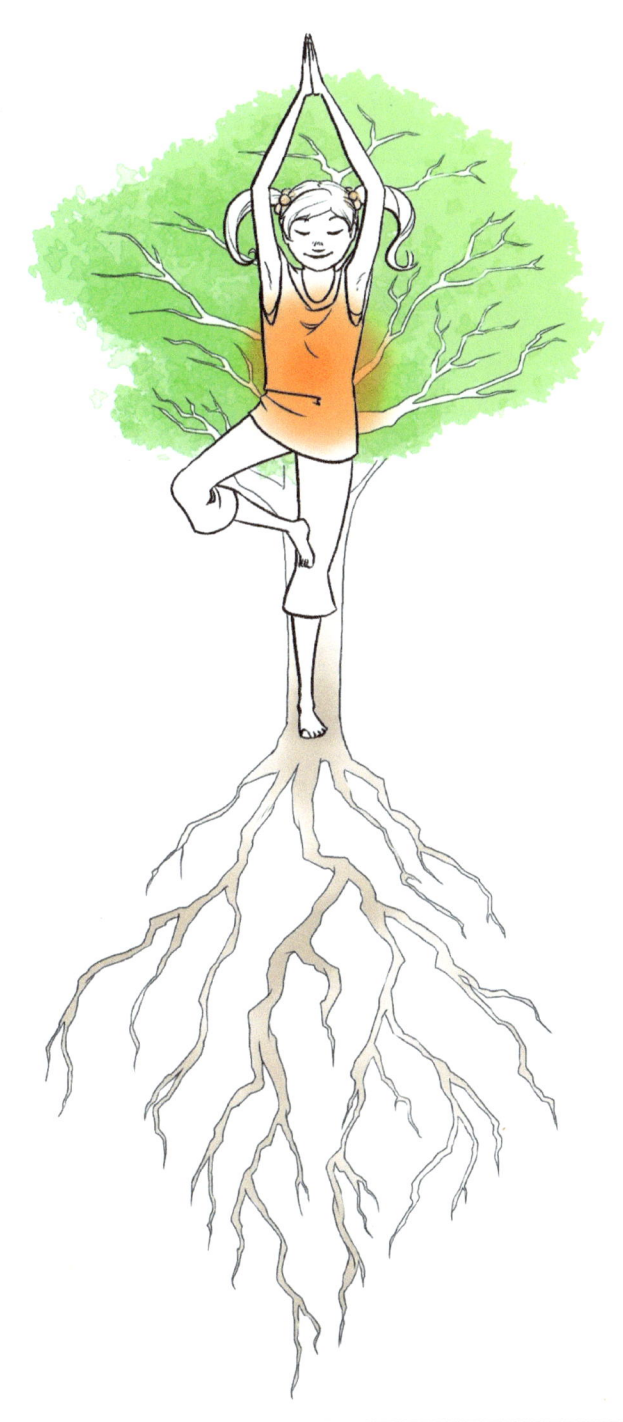

"Now, back to Mountain pose, standing big and tall.
Can you see your nose?"

"Feel peaceful and serene. You just need to breathe.
Let's stop for a moment and feel the heart.
This is the best part!"

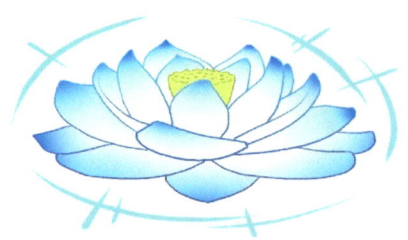

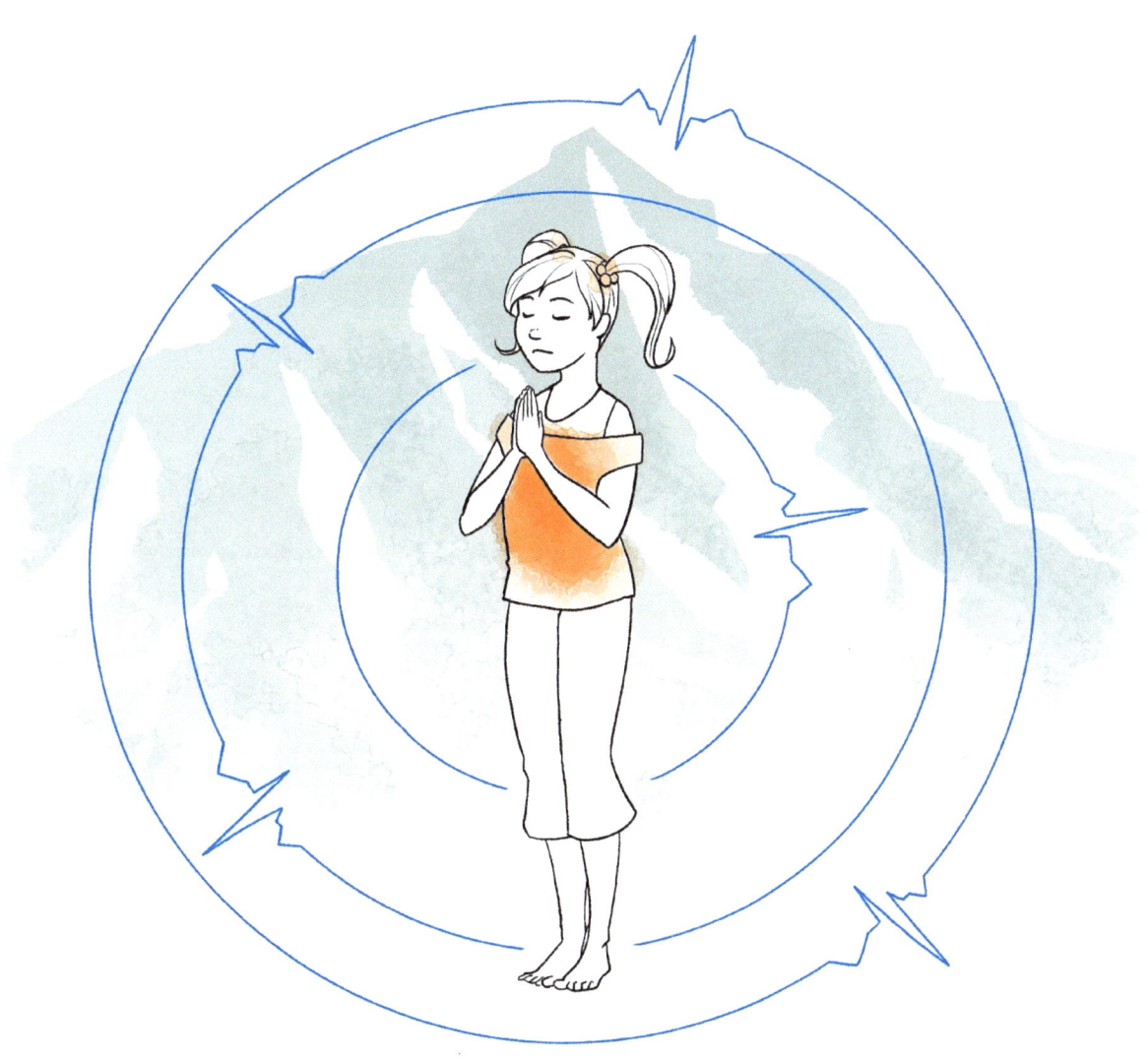

"Come down and sit criss-cross.
This is called easy pose."

Emma and Jake sit quietly for while.

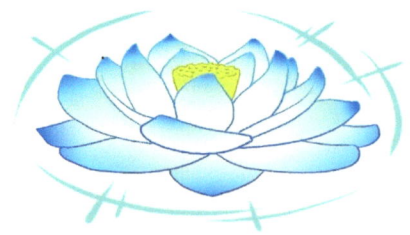

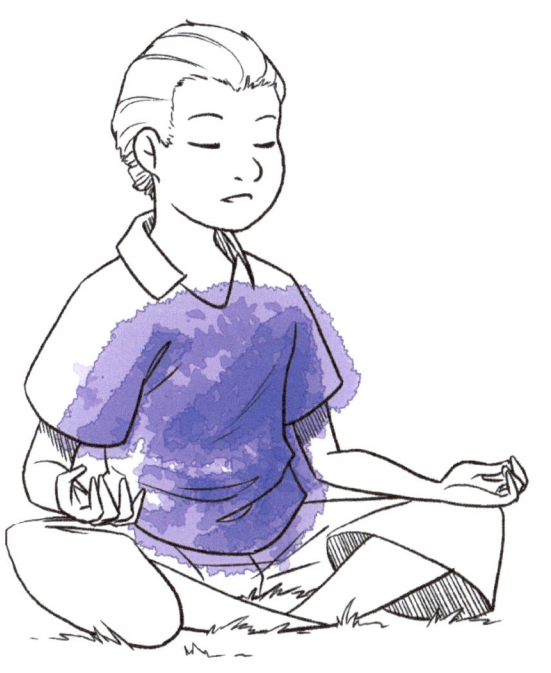
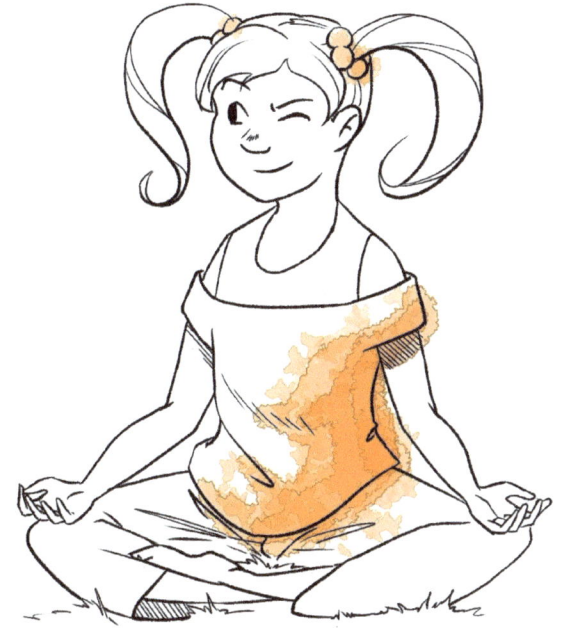

Then Jake opens his eyes with a big smile…
"Thank you" says Jake. "I will do my best to practice
every day."

Emma smiles and says,
"don't forget the loving touch, just use your hands and
send good thoughts."

ALL WE NEED IS LOVE.

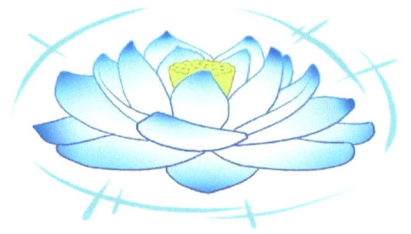

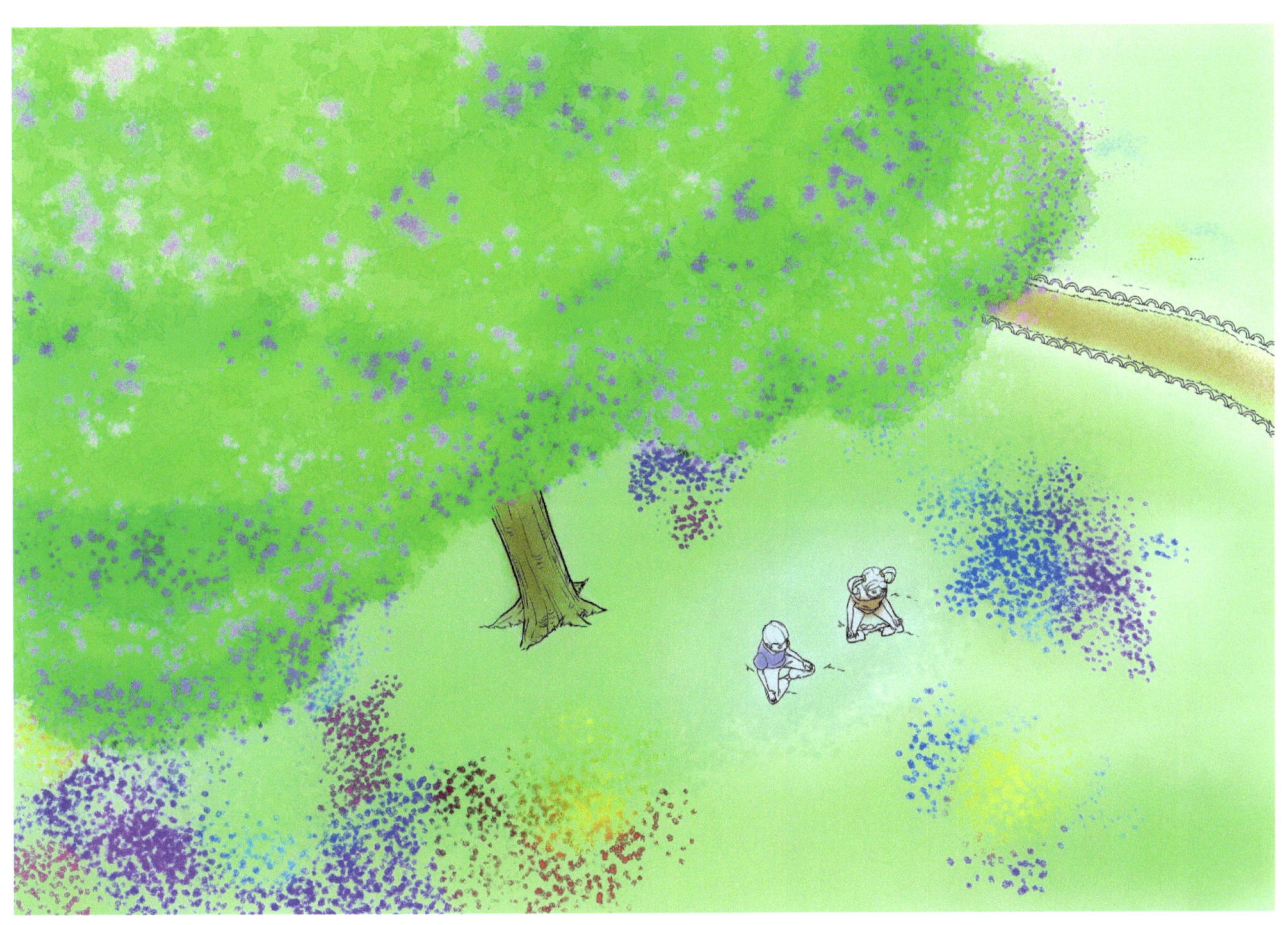

ABOUT THE AUTHOR:

Siomara is a charismatic woman who felt in love with the teachings of yoga and its powerful and transformational tools. She is dedicating her life to bring joy, hope, and inspiration to children and women through the teachings of yoga in combination with other holistic and energy techniques.

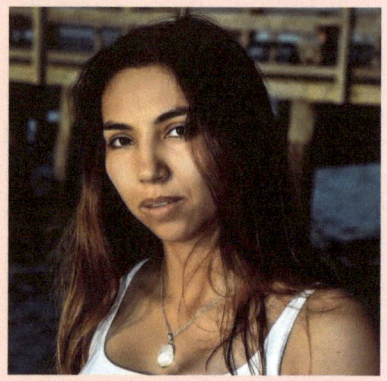

Siomara was born in Colombia in 1981 and found herself truly at home when she moved to NYC at the age of 22. She currently teaches in different private schools in the city, runs women's circles and retreats as well as public classes and private sessions.

Siomara Yogini

For more information you can contact her at
beyou@siomarayogini.com

This book has been edited and designed by John Navidad,
finishing in New York in October, 31, 2017.
There are more books of this and other authors in
www.ManhattanBoundBooks.com

Join our FB Page in:
www.facebook.com/manhattanboundbooks
Contact: JohnNavidadNY@gmail.com